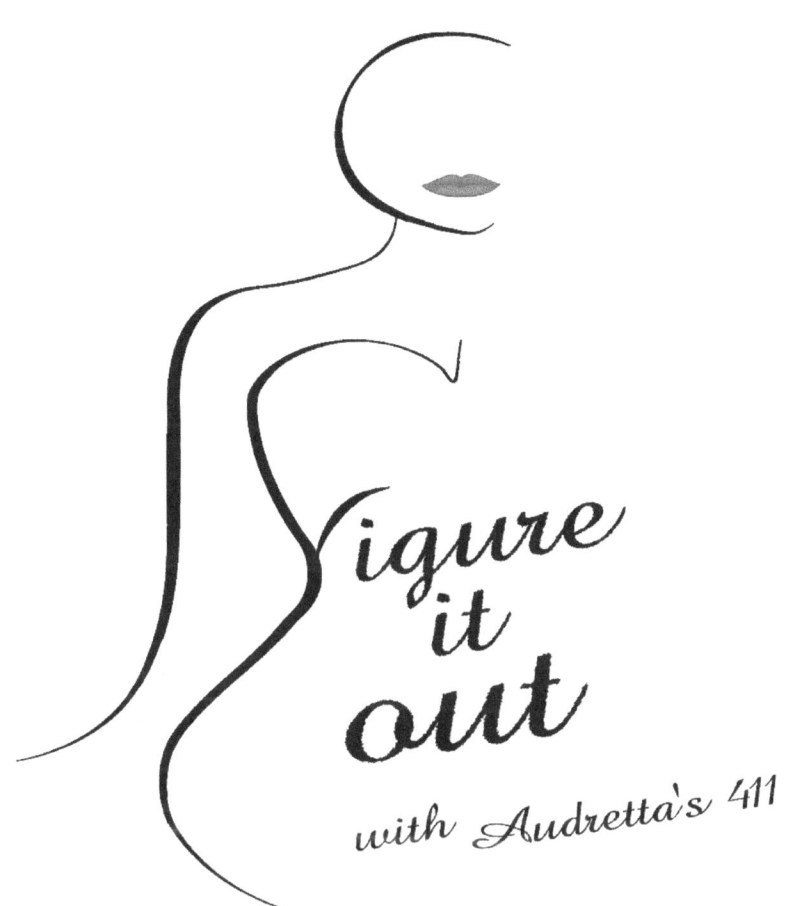

Figure it out

with Audretta's 411

How I lost nearly 100 lbs. when I stopped dieting and Figured OUT the following 7 Eating RULES!

Printed in the United States of America

First Printing, 2018

ISBN-13: 978-1720870166

ISBN-10: 1720870160

Foreward

AT LAST... a book that approaches the subject of weight loss from an emotional and psychological point of view. A mentally interactive tool which subliminally encourages each reader to both examine and reflect upon his or her personal failures (and successes) of the past and provides rarely-thought-of "tips and tricks" to encourage each of us to be proactive in our decision-making as we press forward in our individual journeys towards good health.

Eye-opening and thought provoking "ideas" that will most certainly cause you to strategically think about your destination of success as opposed to being surprised and totally derailed as you encounter the ever-so-unavoidable disappointments along the way.

And most importantly, how to recover a fumble and still win the game!! What an absolutely and utterly refreshing way to approach and view weight loss and health.

--Antionette Randall

"When I met Audretta Hall at a community event, she greeted me with a warm smile and proceeded to share information about the health items she had on the table. She had such a positive energy and confident about her that made me want to stay in touch with her. That was over 10 years ago. Since then, I have gone to several of her events on health and healing, spent personal time with her and lost weight. The pearls of wisdom that Audretta has shared with hundreds and thousands of people regarding healthy lifestyle living has proven to be true and beneficial only if you make use of the information. Over the years of walking this healthy lifestyle journey with my amazing sister in Christ, I have been successful in not only healthy eating habits but also in keeping the extra weight off. While Audretta does encourage you, pray with you, guide you, support you, and love you; not once has she or will she force you to live a healthy lifestyle. The choice is yours and the tools are there if you make use of them. I am very proud of Audretta Hall and I honor her as my friend, my sister in Christ and my health couch! As you take a journey with her in this book and commit to making healthy lifestyle changes, I guarantee you will never be the same and will never allow food or unhealthy habits to take control of your life!"

--Alicia Diggs-Founder of I Will Live

Table of Contents

Eating Rule #1

Family Eating

Old Habit: Eat until you are stuffed and can hardly move!

New Rule: Eat until you are 80% full

(How do you know when you are 80% full? Read on—I will tell you)

Eating in our family, in the old days, was like a sport. Every Holiday we got together there was an unspoken challenge. The Aunts would see who could cook the best food in the largest quantity and the children and Uncles would see who could eat the most. I can remember a Thanksgiving dinner where my Uncle came into the family room with his food on a COOKIE SHEET! Now that is WAY too much food! No wonder our bellies were sticking out. Our shirts didn't stand the chance of touching the tops of our summer shorts! Not good.

As I began my quest to lose weight I learned how detrimental eating until I was completely stuffed was to my health. I have memories of eating so much that I could not lie comfortably on my stomach for an entire DAY! The pressure and the stress this had on my organs had to have been tremendous.

I later learned that my body had been giving me clues of when to stop eating......clues that would have halted my overeating (had I heeded to them) LONG before the pressure had built up.

That deep intake of breath while I was eating was a clue that I was getting full. The weight of the food in your stomach pushes down on your diaphragm causing you to take in a deep breath. That is the body's way of measuring how much food you have in your stomach. The lobe of your lung sits on top of your stomach. If you fill up the space in your stomach, where the lung rest, then you can't take a deep breath! Lord knows I have done this a many a Thanksgiving dinner in my younger 'foolish about health' days. When you eat past this clue you are over taxing your body's digestive system because you are making it process WAY more food than it can in the allotted time period. Your body wants to and must process the food in 2 to 3 hours. Over eating causes your stomach to push food that is not completely processed into the colon. Can you say, 'Big contributor to constipation'?

These days I contribute my successful weight loss to eating until I take that deep breath...I usually have one or two more bites and drink a hot cup of tea. What did that do for me? Well it helped me to go from a size 26 to a size 12!

Read on! There are six more helpful tips. Use them all together or pick a few that work for you. I know that everything is not for everybody and you will only do what you want to do and what comes naturally to you! But these are some of the first steps to help you FIGURE IT OUT!

Action Steps

Time to reflect. Take a minute to write down a few of your thoughts. This will help you to make a personal plan and help you to have written actions steps to figure it out for you!

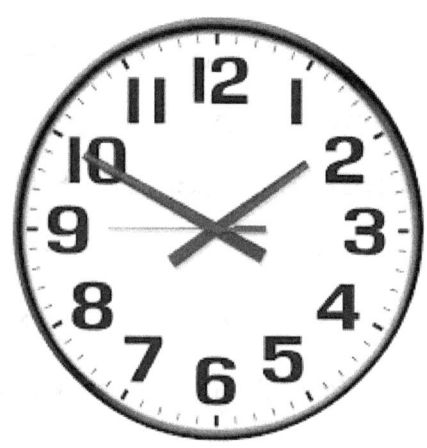

Notes to Self

What did you identify with when reading this chapter?

What was the most useful information?

From what you have now figured out about yourself, which action items can you apply to your daily quest for good health?

List Three things you can share with others after reading this chapter.

Eating Rule #2

Balanced Eating

Old Habit: Wait 8 to 12 hours between meals

New Rule: Eat something healthy every 2 hours in between meals.

I took a page out of the book of observation and noted that skinny people ate all the time! It seemed to me that every skinny person I saw on the street was eating SOMETHING. I, on the other hand, would wait 10 to 12 hours to eat then go put a KILLING on some poor restaurants buffet!

So why was waiting so long to eat such a bad thing for my body? Well I learned that this long-time span without putting any nutrients in my body triggered an ancient instinct that caused my body to go into starvation mode. Basically, my body didn't know when I would eat again so it was turning what I ate in to fat—storing it for emergency purposes. I guess going that long without eating constituted an emergency on the part of my body.

I decided to put my body's mind at rest and eat something healthy every few hours. I snack on almonds, raw carrots, apples. I will have some organic non-GMO popcorn and/or some dark chocolates—just a few. Yes, I said CHOCOLATE. A small amount of dark chocolate seemed to curb my appetite for HOURS after I ate it.

The more often I ate the smaller I got—seriously. I had a sister that joked that I had 'Ate my way to thin'. Well, that was very close to the truth!

Another truth that I learned along the way is that eating more often kept my blood sugar level. My blood sugar would dip so low that I would literally shake. And then I would eat until that shaking feeling went away—and it was not always the BEST of food choices. I can recall a time when I had gone to lunch with co-worker. We were both STARVING. We looked at the menu and both decided on the thing that sounded like a good idea to our starving minds—Blue cheese covered fried potato wedges. That was over 8 years ago and we still laugh at how sick we got eating that day!

By snacking on veggies, like carrots, broccoli & cauliflower, eating these in-between and with meals, I was able to make sensible eating choices when it was time to eat.

Your snack of choice is up to you, but I would not suggest that it be cookies, chips or donuts. These items are high in sugar, calories and have virtually zero nutrients.

Action Steps:

Take a minute and write down what you would enjoy snacking on that will HELP you in your quest to get healthy.

Note to Self

What did you identify with when reading this chapter?

What was the most useful information?

From what you have now figured out about yourself, which action items can you apply to your daily quest for good health?

List Three things you can share with others after reading this chapter.

Eating Rule #3

Drinking and Eating

Old Habit: Drink a ton of cold liquid while eating

New Rule: Don't drink ANYTHING while eating and after eating drink something room temperature or HOT!

Okay, So I was a pretty smart kid in High School. I had graduated at the top of my class and had taken Honor courses in advanced science to boot. So how come it took me so long to figure out that the cold soda that I was drinking with that cheeseburger sub was coagulating the grease in the sub in my system? WOW. No wonder my stomach hurt after that combination of events. Now let's add the fact that I was barely chewing what I ate. When I ate I would take a HUGE bite of what I was eating, chew it a couple of times then rinse the hunk of food down with a gulp of whatever cold liquid I had at the time.

Time was definitely something I wasn't taking! I chewed very little, ate fast and rinsed often. And the rinsing part didn't leave room for what I really needed...chewing! Chewing would have mixed the saliva with my food starting the digestive process where it is supposed to begin—in my mouth! All that food that needed to be softened first ended up in my stomach in one huge ball. I was miserable, bloated and very front tummy heavy (which I hid well because, at 284 lbs, I was a Double F cup—people couldn't even see the size of my belly hidden under THAT shelf!)

I am no longer keeping what I know on a shelf. Now I am telling every that will listen: Use the European Secret to weight loss. Eat light, Eat Right, Eat Often and Drink Hot Tea after a meal. This is the practice in several European countries that are not fighting an epidemic of obesity......being small leaves clues!

Being 14 sizes smaller has definitely taken a bit of getting used to. I have a hard time believing that I am size 10/12 and usually started by trying on pants that a few sizes larger. I am sure I will lose a few more pounds before my 50th Birthday but until then, I can finally say, I am HAPPY with the size that I am right now!

You can vary this rule to fit your needs. Maybe you are a coffee drinker or would like to have some hot soup after a meal. Whichever you prefer is fine with me and, I am almost certain, your body as well.

Notes to Self

What did you identify with when reading this chapter?

What was the most useful information?

From what you have now figured out about yourself, which action items can you apply to your daily quest for good health?

List Three things you can share with others after reading this chapter.

Eating Rule# 4

Get Back in the Saddle

Old Habit: Go off my diet and have a donut? Wait a day, week, month or the next calendar year to get back on track.

New Rule: Get back on track with the NEXT MEAL!

Did that say, 'get back on her diet the next YEAR?' Yeah, and I am almost completely positive that I am not the only one that has done it. In September I would start thinking "I will have to go on my diet after the holidays." Well that IS the next calendar YEAR! I know I was not alone in the thought process of waiting until the next YEAR to get back on my diet. I have been the keynote speaker at several functions and heard this very same mentality voiced quietly amongst the attendees. I would just sigh when I heard it. I had the experience and knowledge to combat that wayward train of thought but would anyone listen and apply the knowledge that I had shared? Would anyone have a donut for breakfast and think ahead enough to just enjoy soup and an apple for lunch?

It does take a bit of "thinking" discipline to get back in the dieting saddle the next meal but you CAN do it. It just takes having a plan. I know WHEN I go off my diet I will have soup, apple and or a salad for the next meal! I also know that my desire for sweets is connected to my hormones being out of balance or my Vitamin D3 level being too low. So when my mind can think of nothing but cheese cake I put some salmon on that salad or take a vitamin D3 supplement! At any rate, either choice has way less calories and can actually help solve the real issue—hormonal imbalance.

Another problem that getting back on track the next meal solves is eliminating the amount of time to gain weight when you have fallen off your dieting horse. I have gained anywhere from 10 to 20 lbs. over the holidays (September to January is 16 weeks... that is gaining just over a pound a week... EASY to do).

I have easily gained and lost about 1,000 lbs. by dieting. I have lost 100 lbs. and kept it off by following the eating rules. Dieting doesn't work for me, counting calories is a nightmare for my mind, and eating bland food drives me to ...EAT MORE! Through trial and error I have figured out what works for me and you can too. Just take a minute to jot down some notes on what you have learned from this chapter. There are no SURPRISE over eating occasions. Thanksgiving is the third Thursday in November, The 4th of July Barb B Que is every... FOURTH OF JULY. Have a plan.

Cut back, walk more and detox the weeks before and you will have a better chance of ENJOYING the occasion. And, you can enjoy the weeks after as well because you will still be able to fit into your pants!

I don't diet at ALL anymore... I figured out what works for me and just follow the eating RULES—RELIGIOUSLY!

Speaking of religion—I have married my faith to my fitness routine! That will be the subject for my next e-book.

In the mean time set yourself up for health and wellness success by having a PLAN for WHEN you get off track. Know the food you are going to eat, how much you are going to eat (One Donut, or THREE Cookies, or ONE slice of pie, or A couple of Slices of pizza) and make sure you get back to nutrient focused eating the next meal.

Here is your chance to write down your plan. Example: Monday Skinny Co-worker brings in Donuts for everyone. Plan—Bring an apple and almonds to snack on before lunch. Have just a sandwich and lemon water for lunch, dark green veggies and a lean meat for dinner.

Remember, No General wins a war by getting up in the morning and saying, "Today I am going to blow up a few bridges, drop a couple of bombs and go home." If you want to win this health war, and you do because you purchased this book, then you have to have a WRITTEN plan!

Action Steps:

Thank yourself for taking a minute to write down your thoughts as a part of your written plan for health success.

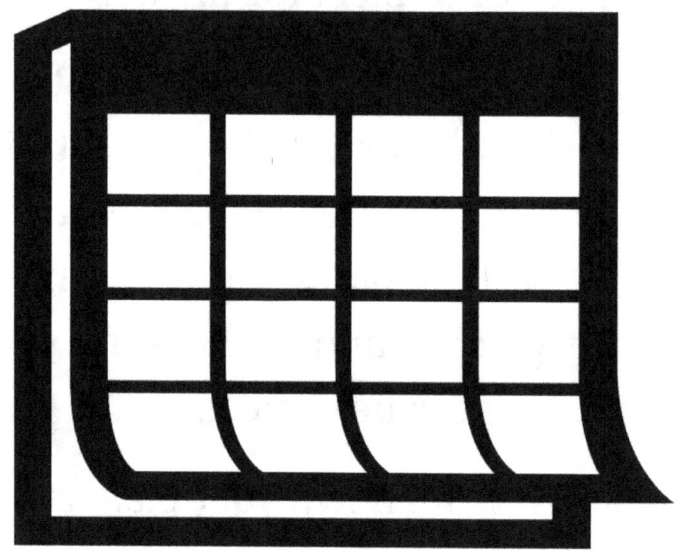

Notes to Self

What did you identify with when reading this chapter?

What was the most useful information?

From what you have now figured out about yourself, which action items can you apply to your daily quest for good health?

List Three things you can share with others after reading this chapter.

Eating Rule #5

Variety: The Key to Good Health

Old Habit: Eat an Entire Box of Cereal or Plate of Spaghetti

New Rule: Eat a small amount of SEVERAL types of food

"When you know better you do better." This is one of the sayings that I got from my mother. I now KNOW better than to sit down on the couch with a bag of potato chips and watch TV. An open bag of chips would be an empty bag of chips in a matter of minutes. I only had to test this theory about 10 times and gain about 15 lbs. before I started to know better.

And knowing better came from putting two and two together while examining my own eating habits. I could open a bag of apples and have just one then why couldn't I open a bag of chips and have just one? I could open a bag of carrots and just eat a couple then why couldn't I open a bag of cookies and have just a couple? I decided to have the apple or carrot BEFORE the chips and or cookie and low and behold, when I did just that, I could stop eating the undesirable food before it got to the end of the bag!

I am now a BAG LADY! When I go to the grocery store I get a bag of apples, a bag of oranges, a bag of carrots and bag of celery! I used to get a bag of cookies, a bag of chips and bag... changing my bag reduced my sag!

My goal at each meal is to reduce blandness. By introducing a variety of foods, flavors and texture I swear my mind and body enjoy the dining experience even more. I used to have about 10 slices of pizza, chips and soda. Now I have two slices with a green salad (spinach leaves, strawberries, red onions almonds with a raspberry vinaigrette dressing) an apple and a glass of water! Eating this way allows me to A.C.E my meal—getting Vitamin A, C and E from the accompanying foods! I do believe that the nutrients are what kept my mind from going into a feeding frenzy. I am totally satisfied at the end of the meal and the scale is totally happy with the results at the end of the week.

Everyone knows what you need to do to lose weight. The real trick comes in how not to gain it. Adding fruits and vegetables to my diet decreased the amount of chemically laden foods in my diet and gave my body the nutrients it needed to properly use the food it was getting.

I am not sure if this will work for you. Try getting a variety in... instead of an entire plate of spaghetti or a whole box of cereal. Eat a bowl of cereal, with an apple, piece of toast and some juice. You get the idea. And this idea will help you figure it out for YOU!

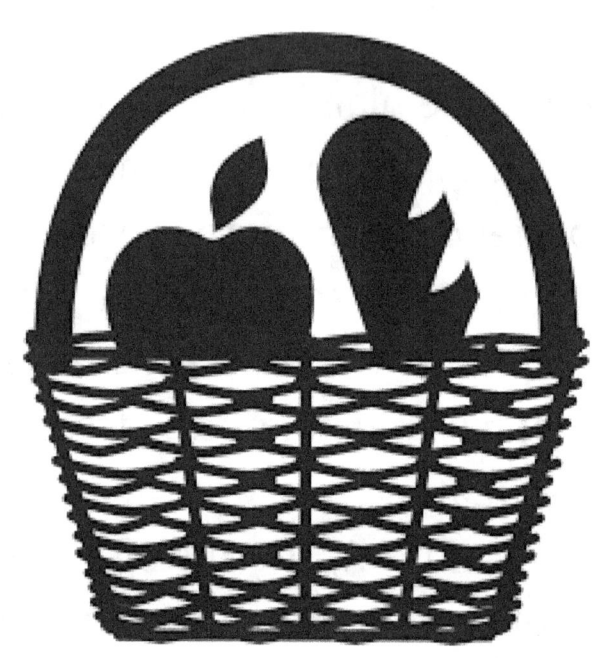

Notes to Self

What did you identify with when reading this chapter?

What was the most useful information?

From what you have now figured out about yourself, which action items can you apply to your daily quest for good health?

List Three things you can share with others after reading this chapter.

Eating Rule #6

The Numbers Game

Old Habit: Counting Calories

New Rule: Count Fiber, Protein, Sugar, Sodium

I cannot tell you how much weight I GAINED trying to count calories—20, 30 pounds? Okay, not all of it was the calorie counting diets fault. I take the blame! I just couldn't or wouldn't count all the calories. For example: I would make a peanut butter and jelly sandwich. The jar said that one tablespoon of peanut butter was 90 calories. I would put two spoons of peanut butter on the bread and 2 or 3 spoons in my mouth. Now I only counted the peanut butter that made it to the bread. The SCALE counted BOTH! I am not sure if that example was a "wouldn't" or a "couldn't" but either way you slice it I was still getting bigger!

I had a big challenge counting calories at restaurants, keeping up with the calories consumed when snacking. I had a personal trainer tell me that if I got 100 grams of protein in a day that I would lose weight naturally. Miraculously something switched in my brain and the focus went on getting protein in and I started making different food choices, quit counting calories and started losing weight.

So what other gems was I missing by focusing only on counting calories? I started snooping around the internet and learned that the average American diet only has 7 to 9 grams of fiber and the average Chinese diet has about 50 to 70 grams of fiber. Now which culture is healthier? Yeah... My thoughts exactly. That is when I started playing the numbers game... with a different set of numbers in mind. Old Habit— concentrate on calorie restriction. New rule: GET IT IN! 40 grams of fiber, 100 grams of protein keep sodium to less than 850mg and sugar to 75 grams or less (had to up the sugar thing because I LOVE juice).

Now these numbers may vary for you depending on your age and lifestyle. Ask your physician or dietician to give you the recommended amounts of fiber, protein, sodium and salt that fits YOU!

And YOU are who this needs to work for. Taylor it to fit your schedule, your health and wellness goals and what works for you! If counting calories is working for you... don't change it. I am not here to reinvent the health and wellness wheel. I am just here to rotate a tire or two to help you get better results.

Notes to Self

What did you identify with when reading this chapter?

What was the most useful information?

From what you have now figured out about yourself, which action items can you apply to your daily quest for good health?

List Three things you can share with others after reading this chapter.

I can't even pronounce that

Old Habit: Eat Anything

New Rule: Only eat things that are preservative, GMO free and with no more than FIVE ingredients

Now read this very slowly and a few times if you have to. When I started doing this—eating as chemical free as humanly possible—I lost weight so fast people thought that I was doing DRUGS! Apparently when that comedian said, "I'm not fat... I'm just SWOLE" it was funny but also 90% true. For me, chemicals in the foods I ate had caused internal swelling and that swelling was telling my body to store and make fat to protect itself.

Fat storage avoidance became my primary goal. I read the back of everything and if it had more than five ingredients in it... I didn't eat it. Margarine was the FIRST thing to go. I read the list of things it had in it and never purchased another tub of the stuff. Now butter, on the other hand, was all the way cool. The label just said, milk, cream and salt. It made the list. So did Breyer's ice cream... I just have to do it in moderation and eat some fresh strawberries with it (A.C.E My meal.)

Here are just a few of my before and after photos. I had been over 200 lbs since I was 18 years old. It has taken me 10 years to reach my goal weight and I have shared with you what has helped me to achieve that goal. I guess I will write about how I got that un-healthy in the next e-book!

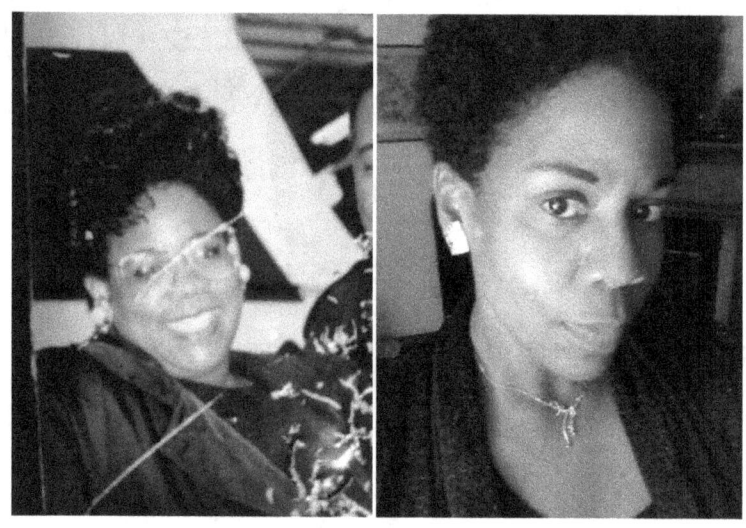

1992   age 27   2014   age 49

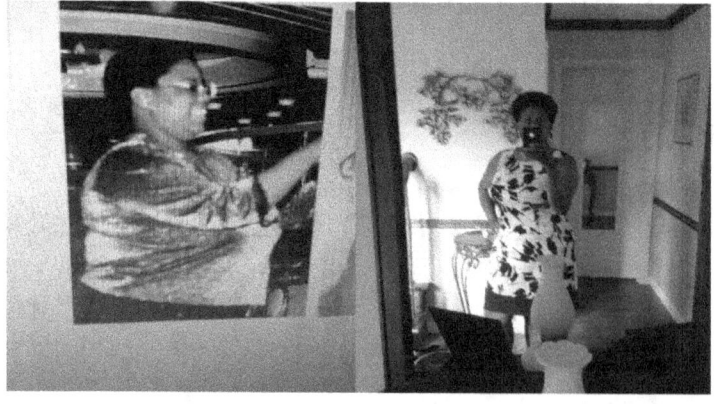

1998 age 33   2014   age 49

Notes to Self

What did you identify with when reading this chapter?

What was the most useful information?

From what you have now figured out about yourself, which action items can you apply to your daily quest for good health?

List Three things you can share with others after reading this chapter.

Bonus: Power Eating Strategies

1. No Surprise over eating occasions- PREPARE! Thanksgiving is the third Thursday in November—EVERY YEAR. So, in October I increase my fiber to 25 to 40 grams a day, eat 100 grams a day of protein, drink detox tea and walk 30 minutes a day. I usually drop 10 to 15lbs BEFORE Thanksgiving—gain five pounds back. But, that means I start The New Year off 5 to 10lbs LIGHTER than the Year Before!

2. Make a Decision of what I am going to eat BEFORE I get hungry. "The next time I get hungry I am going to have...an apple and some yogurt."

3. Don't concentrate on everything at once. Go 10 days without fried food. Then 10 days no sweets. Then 10 days no sodas or sweet teas. Then 10 days working out EVERYDAY. Then 10 days low salt. Then 10 days drinking 64 oz plus of water... you get the picture. When I did everything at once it left nothing to shock the body with...thus I would hit a plateau and have nothing left to!

4. Eat things that reduces inflammation and swelling in the body. Swelling TELLS your body to store and make FAT.

5. EAT a ton of Onions, spices, garlic, olive oil, coconut oil, cilantro, basil, rosemary, thymes, turmeric etc. because it helps to reduce inflammation, parasite and yeast. Both are

a source of swelling in the body and, again, swelling tells the body to store and make fat.

6. Get the right amount of nutrients through supplements. D3 & Selenium Helps control your hormones, Magnesium helps control migraines and period pain, Potassium reduces blood pressure and body cramps, calcium and Co-Que 10 helps the body maintain a balanced weight.

7. Eat a variety of FOODS that contain the nutrients you need. Supplementation means just that... take in ADDITION to... not in replace OF.

8. Hydrate and do everything you can to reduce inflammation in your body. Don't eat foods that cause you to swell. Swelling tells your body to store and make fat to protect itself.

For more information on inflammation reducing foods, spices and health tips in general visit my Facebook page at www.facebook.com/transformationaudrettas411

For a personal consultation please email me at Audrettas411@gmail.com and I will send you a brief questionnaire and, together we can work on a plan that FIGURES IT out for YOU!

Reference Page

Vitamin D information	www.everydayhealth.com
Fiber Facts	www.mayoclinic.org
Fight Inflammation	www.liverdoctor.com

About The Author

Raised in a large family steeped in the traditions of over eating, Audretta Hall was introduced to the concept that indulging in rich decadent foods in large quantities meant "love". By the age of 10, Audretta was over 130lbs. and by the age of 18 she was well over 200 lbs. on a 5'7" frame.

Despite going on numerous diets and taking countless potions and pills, Audretta Continued to gain weight during her college years. Audretta hit an academic mile stone when she received a degree in Advertising from Michigan State University and hit physical pinnacle of 225lbs!

College stress eating triggered a 20lbs weight gain. Marriage stress along with GOOD times eating led to another 60 lbs. of stored fat.

By the end of Audretta's first marriage, Audretta was over 280lbs. and seriously looking for answers to her weight gain. Knowing that she was just single digit pounds away from tipping she scale to the 300lbs. mark Audretta began searching internet, God and herself for health success and clues.

Audretta put The Bible in the kitchen and began to read upon entering the kitchen. This simple trick gave her the strength to eat just a couple of Oreo cookies... instead of an entire sleeve.

This simple act, using her faith helped Audretta to lose her first 15lbs.

With that weight loss success, Audretta was inspired to try non-traditional methods, things out side of diet and exercising. Two things that had not worked for her.

In the pages of this work book the reader will find what Audretta Figured OUT during her quest with each chapter accompanied by a "what did I learn" section for each reader to fill out. In doing so, every reader of "Figure it OUT with Audretta's 411" will have the beginnings of their own personal health and wellness plan.

Creating a personalized health and wellness plan can be a simple process when you pair it with daily tips and coaching. Join Audretta's 411 Facebook and you can receive tips on a daily/weekly basis.

Visit www.facebook.com/transformationaudrettas411 to receive a free 30-minute consultation please send an email with your name, phone number and two good times to call to audrettas411@gmail.com.

Read, Write, Gain INSIGHT and FIGURE IT OUT!

www.ingramcontent.com/pod-product-compliance
Lightning Source LLC
Chambersburg PA
CBHW081648220526
45468CB00009B/2585